The Heart Failure Patient Log

DATE:

BP:

WEIGHT:

GLUCOSE:

SYMPTOMS:

DATE:

BP:

WEIGHT:

GLUCOSE:

SYMPTOMS:

DATE:

BP:

WEIGHT:

GLUCOSE:

SYMPTOMS:

DATE:

BP:

WEIGHT:

GLUCOSE:

SYMPTOMS:

DATE:

BP:

WEIGHT:

GLUCOSE:

SYMPTOMS:

DATE:

BP:

WEIGHT:

GLUCOSE:

SYMPTOMS:

DATE:

BP:

WEIGHT:

GLUCOSE:

SYMPTOMS:

DATE:

BP:

WEIGHT:

GLUCOSE:

SYMPTOMS:

DATE:

BP:

WEIGHT:

GLUCOSE:

SYMPTOMS:

DATE:

BP:

WEIGHT:

GLUCOSE:

SYMPTOMS:

DATE:

BP:

WEIGHT:

GLUCOSE:

SYMPTOMS:

DATE:

BP:

WEIGHT:

GLUCOSE:

SYMPTOMS:

DATE:

BP:

WEIGHT:

GLUCOSE:

SYMPTOMS:

DATE:

BP:

WEIGHT:

GLUCOSE:

SYMPTOMS:

DATE:

BP:

WEIGHT:

GLUCOSE:

SYMPTOMS:

DATE:

BP:

WEIGHT:

GLUCOSE:

SYMPTOMS:

DATE:

BP:

WEIGHT:

GLUCOSE:

SYMPTOMS:

DATE:

BP:

WEIGHT:

GLUCOSE:

SYMPTOMS:

DATE:

BP:

WEIGHT:

GLUCOSE:

SYMPTOMS:

DATE:

BP:

WEIGHT:

GLUCOSE:

SYMPTOMS:

DATE:

BP:

WEIGHT:

GLUCOSE:

SYMPTOMS:

DATE:

BP:

WEIGHT:

GLUCOSE:

SYMPTOMS:

DATE:

BP:

WEIGHT:

GLUCOSE:

SYMPTOMS:

DATE:

BP:

WEIGHT:

GLUCOSE:

SYMPTOMS:

DATE:

BP:

WEIGHT:

GLUCOSE:

SYMPTOMS:

DATE:

BP:

WEIGHT:

GLUCOSE:

SYMPTOMS:

DATE:

BP:

WEIGHT:

GLUCOSE:

SYMPTOMS:

DATE:

BP:

WEIGHT:

GLUCOSE:

SYMPTOMS:

DATE:

BP:

WEIGHT:

GLUCOSE:

SYMPTOMS:

DATE:

BP:

WEIGHT:

GLUCOSE:

SYMPTOMS:

DATE:

BP:

WEIGHT:

GLUCOSE:

SYMPTOMS:

DATE:

BP:

WEIGHT:

GLUCOSE:

SYMPTOMS:

DATE:

BP:

WEIGHT:

GLUCOSE:

SYMPTOMS:

DATE:

BP:

WEIGHT:

GLUCOSE:

SYMPTOMS:

DATE:

BP:

WEIGHT:

GLUCOSE:

SYMPTOMS:

DATE:

BP:

WEIGHT:

GLUCOSE:

SYMPTOMS:

DATE:

BP:

WEIGHT:

GLUCOSE:

SYMPTOMS:

DATE:

BP:

WEIGHT:

GLUCOSE:

SYMPTOMS:

DATE:

BP:

WEIGHT:

GLUCOSE:

SYMPTOMS:

DATE:

BP:

WEIGHT:

GLUCOSE:

SYMPTOMS:

DATE:

BP:

WEIGHT:

GLUCOSE:

SYMPTOMS:

DATE:

BP:

WEIGHT:

GLUCOSE:

SYMPTOMS:

DATE:

BP:

WEIGHT:

GLUCOSE:

SYMPTOMS:

DATE:

BP:

WEIGHT:

GLUCOSE:

SYMPTOMS:

DATE:

BP:

WEIGHT:

GLUCOSE:

SYMPTOMS:

DATE:

BP:

WEIGHT:

GLUCOSE:

SYMPTOMS:

DATE:

BP:

WEIGHT:

GLUCOSE:

SYMPTOMS:

DATE:

BP:

WEIGHT:

GLUCOSE:

SYMPTOMS:

DATE:

BP:

WEIGHT:

GLUCOSE:

SYMPTOMS:

DATE:

BP:

WEIGHT:

GLUCOSE:

SYMPTOMS:

DATE:

BP:

WEIGHT:

GLUCOSE:

SYMPTOMS:

DATE:

BP:

WEIGHT:

GLUCOSE:

SYMPTOMS:

DATE:

BP:

WEIGHT:

GLUCOSE:

SYMPTOMS:

DATE:

BP:

WEIGHT:

GLUCOSE:

SYMPTOMS:

DATE:

BP:

WEIGHT:

GLUCOSE:

SYMPTOMS:

DATE:

BP:

WEIGHT:

GLUCOSE:

SYMPTOMS:

DATE:

BP:

WEIGHT:

GLUCOSE:

SYMPTOMS:

DATE:

BP:

WEIGHT:

GLUCOSE:

SYMPTOMS:

DATE:

BP:

WEIGHT:

GLUCOSE:

SYMPTOMS:

DATE:

BP:

WEIGHT:

GLUCOSE:

SYMPTOMS:

DATE:

BP:

WEIGHT:

GLUCOSE:

SYMPTOMS:

DATE:

BP:

WEIGHT:

GLUCOSE:

SYMPTOMS:

DATE:

BP:

WEIGHT:

GLUCOSE:

SYMPTOMS:

DATE:

BP:

WEIGHT:

GLUCOSE:

SYMPTOMS:

DATE:

BP:

WEIGHT:

GLUCOSE:

SYMPTOMS:

DATE:

BP:

WEIGHT:

GLUCOSE:

SYMPTOMS:

DATE:

BP:

WEIGHT:

GLUCOSE:

SYMPTOMS:

DATE:

BP:

WEIGHT:

GLUCOSE:

SYMPTOMS:

DATE:

BP:

WEIGHT:

GLUCOSE:

SYMPTOMS:

DATE:

BP:

WEIGHT:

GLUCOSE:

SYMPTOMS:

DATE:

BP:

WEIGHT:

GLUCOSE:

SYMPTOMS:

DATE:

BP:

WEIGHT:

GLUCOSE:

SYMPTOMS:

DATE:

BP:

WEIGHT:

GLUCOSE:

SYMPTOMS:

DATE:

BP:

WEIGHT:

GLUCOSE:

SYMPTOMS:

DATE:

BP:

WEIGHT:

GLUCOSE:

SYMPTOMS:

DATE:

BP:

WEIGHT:

GLUCOSE:

SYMPTOMS:

DATE:

BP:

WEIGHT:

GLUCOSE:

SYMPTOMS:

DATE:

BP:

WEIGHT:

GLUCOSE:

SYMPTOMS:

DATE:

BP:

WEIGHT:

GLUCOSE:

SYMPTOMS:

DATE:

BP:

WEIGHT:

GLUCOSE:

SYMPTOMS:

DATE:

BP:

WEIGHT:

GLUCOSE:

SYMPTOMS:

DATE:

BP:

WEIGHT:

GLUCOSE:

SYMPTOMS:

DATE:

BP:

WEIGHT:

GLUCOSE:

SYMPTOMS:

DATE:

BP:

WEIGHT:

GLUCOSE:

SYMPTOMS:

DATE:

BP:

WEIGHT:

GLUCOSE:

SYMPTOMS:

DATE:

BP:

WEIGHT:

GLUCOSE:

SYMPTOMS:

DATE:

BP:

WEIGHT:

GLUCOSE:

SYMPTOMS:

DATE:

BP:

WEIGHT:

GLUCOSE:

SYMPTOMS:

DATE:

BP:

WEIGHT:

GLUCOSE:

SYMPTOMS:

DATE:

BP:

WEIGHT:

GLUCOSE:

SYMPTOMS:

DATE:

BP:

WEIGHT:

GLUCOSE:

SYMPTOMS:

DATE:

BP:

WEIGHT:

GLUCOSE:

SYMPTOMS:

DATE:

BP:

WEIGHT:

GLUCOSE:

SYMPTOMS:

DATE:

BP:

WEIGHT:

GLUCOSE:

SYMPTOMS:

DATE:

BP:

WEIGHT:

GLUCOSE:

SYMPTOMS:

DATE:

BP:

WEIGHT:

GLUCOSE:

SYMPTOMS:

DATE:

BP:

WEIGHT:

GLUCOSE:

SYMPTOMS:

DATE:

BP:

WEIGHT:

GLUCOSE:

SYMPTOMS:

DATE:

BP:

WEIGHT:

GLUCOSE:

SYMPTOMS:

DATE:

BP:

WEIGHT:

GLUCOSE:

SYMPTOMS:

DATE:

BP:

WEIGHT:

GLUCOSE:

SYMPTOMS:

DATE:

BP:

WEIGHT:

GLUCOSE:

SYMPTOMS:

DATE:

BP:

WEIGHT:

GLUCOSE:

SYMPTOMS:

DATE:

BP:

WEIGHT:

GLUCOSE:

SYMPTOMS:

DATE:

BP:

WEIGHT:

GLUCOSE:

SYMPTOMS:

DATE:

BP:

WEIGHT:

GLUCOSE:

SYMPTOMS:

DATE:

BP:

WEIGHT:

GLUCOSE:

SYMPTOMS:

DATE:

BP:

WEIGHT:

GLUCOSE:

SYMPTOMS:

DATE:

BP:

WEIGHT:

GLUCOSE:

SYMPTOMS:

DATE:

BP:

WEIGHT:

GLUCOSE:

SYMPTOMS:

DATE:

BP:

WEIGHT:

GLUCOSE:

SYMPTOMS:

DATE:

BP:

WEIGHT:

GLUCOSE:

SYMPTOMS:

DATE:

BP:

WEIGHT:

GLUCOSE:

SYMPTOMS:

DATE:

BP:

WEIGHT:

GLUCOSE:

SYMPTOMS:

DATE:

BP:

WEIGHT:

GLUCOSE:

SYMPTOMS:

DATE:

BP:

WEIGHT:

GLUCOSE:

SYMPTOMS:

DATE:

BP:

WEIGHT:

GLUCOSE:

SYMPTOMS:

DATE:

BP:

WEIGHT:

GLUCOSE:

SYMPTOMS:

DATE:

BP:

WEIGHT:

GLUCOSE:

SYMPTOMS:

DATE:

BP:

WEIGHT:

GLUCOSE:

SYMPTOMS:

DATE:

BP:

WEIGHT:

GLUCOSE:

SYMPTOMS:

DATE:

BP:

WEIGHT:

GLUCOSE:

SYMPTOMS:

DATE:

BP:

WEIGHT:

GLUCOSE:

SYMPTOMS:

DATE:

BP:

WEIGHT:

GLUCOSE:

SYMPTOMS:

DATE:

BP:

WEIGHT:

GLUCOSE:

SYMPTOMS:

DATE:

BP:

WEIGHT:

GLUCOSE:

SYMPTOMS:

DATE:

BP:

WEIGHT:

GLUCOSE:

SYMPTOMS:

DATE:

BP:

WEIGHT:

GLUCOSE:

SYMPTOMS:

DATE:

BP:

WEIGHT:

GLUCOSE:

SYMPTOMS:

DATE:

BP:

WEIGHT:

GLUCOSE:

SYMPTOMS:

DATE:

BP:

WEIGHT:

GLUCOSE:

SYMPTOMS:

DATE:

BP:

WEIGHT:

GLUCOSE:

SYMPTOMS:

DATE:

BP:

WEIGHT:

GLUCOSE:

SYMPTOMS:

DATE:

BP:

WEIGHT:

GLUCOSE:

SYMPTOMS:

DATE:

BP:

WEIGHT:

GLUCOSE:

SYMPTOMS:

DATE:

BP:

WEIGHT:

GLUCOSE:

SYMPTOMS:

DATE:

BP:

WEIGHT:

GLUCOSE:

SYMPTOMS:

DATE:

BP:

WEIGHT:

GLUCOSE:

SYMPTOMS:

DATE:

BP:

WEIGHT:

GLUCOSE:

SYMPTOMS:

DATE:

BP:

WEIGHT:

GLUCOSE:

SYMPTOMS:

DATE:

BP:

WEIGHT:

GLUCOSE:

SYMPTOMS:

DATE:

BP:

WEIGHT:

GLUCOSE:

SYMPTOMS:

DATE:

BP:

WEIGHT:

GLUCOSE:

SYMPTOMS:

DATE:

BP:

WEIGHT:

GLUCOSE:

SYMPTOMS:

DATE:

BP:

WEIGHT:

GLUCOSE:

SYMPTOMS:

DATE:

BP:

WEIGHT:

GLUCOSE:

SYMPTOMS:

DATE:

BP:

WEIGHT:

GLUCOSE:

SYMPTOMS:

DATE:

BP:

WEIGHT:

GLUCOSE:

SYMPTOMS:

DATE:

BP:

WEIGHT:

GLUCOSE:

SYMPTOMS:

DATE:

BP:

WEIGHT:

GLUCOSE:

SYMPTOMS:

DATE:

BP:

WEIGHT:

GLUCOSE:

SYMPTOMS:

DATE:

BP:

WEIGHT:

GLUCOSE:

SYMPTOMS:

DATE:

BP:

WEIGHT:

GLUCOSE:

SYMPTOMS:

DATE:

BP:

WEIGHT:

GLUCOSE:

SYMPTOMS:

DATE:

BP:

WEIGHT:

GLUCOSE:

SYMPTOMS:

DATE:

BP:

WEIGHT:

GLUCOSE:

SYMPTOMS:

DATE:

BP:

WEIGHT:

GLUCOSE:

SYMPTOMS:

DATE:

BP:

WEIGHT:

GLUCOSE:

SYMPTOMS:

DATE:

BP:

WEIGHT:

GLUCOSE:

SYMPTOMS:

DATE:

BP:

WEIGHT:

GLUCOSE:

SYMPTOMS:

DATE:

BP:

WEIGHT:

GLUCOSE:

SYMPTOMS:

DATE:

BP:

WEIGHT:

GLUCOSE:

SYMPTOMS:

DATE:

BP:

WEIGHT:

GLUCOSE:

SYMPTOMS:

DATE:

BP:

WEIGHT:

GLUCOSE:

SYMPTOMS:

DATE:

BP:

WEIGHT:

GLUCOSE:

SYMPTOMS:

DATE:

BP:

WEIGHT:

GLUCOSE:

SYMPTOMS:

DATE:

BP:

WEIGHT:

GLUCOSE:

SYMPTOMS:

DATE:

BP:

WEIGHT:

GLUCOSE:

SYMPTOMS:

DATE:

BP:

WEIGHT:

GLUCOSE:

SYMPTOMS:

DATE:

BP:

WEIGHT:

GLUCOSE:

SYMPTOMS:

DATE:

BP:

WEIGHT:

GLUCOSE:

SYMPTOMS:

DATE:

BP:

WEIGHT:

GLUCOSE:

SYMPTOMS:

DATE:

BP:

WEIGHT:

GLUCOSE:

SYMPTOMS:

DATE:

BP:

WEIGHT:

GLUCOSE:

SYMPTOMS:

DATE:

BP:

WEIGHT:

GLUCOSE:

SYMPTOMS:

DATE:

BP:

WEIGHT:

GLUCOSE:

SYMPTOMS:

DATE:

BP:

WEIGHT:

GLUCOSE:

SYMPTOMS:

DATE:

BP:

WEIGHT:

GLUCOSE:

SYMPTOMS:

DATE:

BP:

WEIGHT:

GLUCOSE:

SYMPTOMS:

DATE:

BP:

WEIGHT:

GLUCOSE:

SYMPTOMS:

DATE:

BP:

WEIGHT:

GLUCOSE:

SYMPTOMS:

DATE:

BP:

WEIGHT:

GLUCOSE:

SYMPTOMS:

DATE:

BP:

WEIGHT:

GLUCOSE:

SYMPTOMS:

DATE:

BP:

WEIGHT:

GLUCOSE:

SYMPTOMS:

DATE:

BP:

WEIGHT:

GLUCOSE:

SYMPTOMS:

DATE:

BP:

WEIGHT:

GLUCOSE:

SYMPTOMS:

DATE:

BP:

WEIGHT:

GLUCOSE:

SYMPTOMS:

DATE:

BP:

WEIGHT:

GLUCOSE:

SYMPTOMS:

DATE:

BP:

WEIGHT:

GLUCOSE:

SYMPTOMS:

DATE:

BP:

WEIGHT:

GLUCOSE:

SYMPTOMS:

DATE:

BP:

WEIGHT:

GLUCOSE:

SYMPTOMS:

DATE:

BP:

WEIGHT:

GLUCOSE:

SYMPTOMS:

DATE:

BP:

WEIGHT:

GLUCOSE:

SYMPTOMS:

DATE:

BP:

WEIGHT:

GLUCOSE:

SYMPTOMS:

DATE:

BP:

WEIGHT:

GLUCOSE:

SYMPTOMS:

DATE:

BP:

WEIGHT:

GLUCOSE:

SYMPTOMS:

DATE:

BP:

WEIGHT:

GLUCOSE:

SYMPTOMS:

DATE:

BP:

WEIGHT:

GLUCOSE:

SYMPTOMS:

DATE:

BP:

WEIGHT:

GLUCOSE:

SYMPTOMS:

DATE:

BP:

WEIGHT:

GLUCOSE:

SYMPTOMS:

DATE:

BP:

WEIGHT:

GLUCOSE:

SYMPTOMS:

DATE:

BP:

WEIGHT:

GLUCOSE:

SYMPTOMS:

DATE:

BP:

WEIGHT:

GLUCOSE:

SYMPTOMS:

DATE:

BP:

WEIGHT:

GLUCOSE:

SYMPTOMS:

DATE:

BP:

WEIGHT:

GLUCOSE:

SYMPTOMS:

DATE:

BP:

WEIGHT:

GLUCOSE:

SYMPTOMS:

DATE:

BP:

WEIGHT:

GLUCOSE:

SYMPTOMS:

DATE:

BP:

WEIGHT:

GLUCOSE:

SYMPTOMS:

DATE:

BP:

WEIGHT:

GLUCOSE:

SYMPTOMS:

DATE:

BP:

WEIGHT:

GLUCOSE:

SYMPTOMS:

DATE:

BP:

WEIGHT:

GLUCOSE:

SYMPTOMS:

DATE:

BP:

WEIGHT:

GLUCOSE:

SYMPTOMS:

DATE:

BP:

WEIGHT:

GLUCOSE:

SYMPTOMS:

DATE:

BP:

WEIGHT:

GLUCOSE:

SYMPTOMS:

DATE:

BP:

WEIGHT:

GLUCOSE:

SYMPTOMS:

DATE:

BP:

WEIGHT:

GLUCOSE:

SYMPTOMS:

DATE:

BP:

WEIGHT:

GLUCOSE:

SYMPTOMS:

DATE:

BP:

WEIGHT:

GLUCOSE:

SYMPTOMS:

DATE:

BP:

WEIGHT:

GLUCOSE:

SYMPTOMS:

DATE:

BP:

WEIGHT:

GLUCOSE:

SYMPTOMS:

DATE:

BP:

WEIGHT:

GLUCOSE:

SYMPTOMS:

DATE:

BP:

WEIGHT:

GLUCOSE:

SYMPTOMS:

DATE:

BP:

WEIGHT:

GLUCOSE:

SYMPTOMS:

DATE:

BP:

WEIGHT:

GLUCOSE:

SYMPTOMS:

DATE:

BP:

WEIGHT:

GLUCOSE:

SYMPTOMS:

DATE:

BP:

WEIGHT:

GLUCOSE:

SYMPTOMS:

DATE:

BP:

WEIGHT:

GLUCOSE:

SYMPTOMS:

DATE:

BP:

WEIGHT:

GLUCOSE:

SYMPTOMS:

DATE:

BP:

WEIGHT:

GLUCOSE:

SYMPTOMS:

DATE:

BP:

WEIGHT:

GLUCOSE:

SYMPTOMS:

DATE:

BP:

WEIGHT:

GLUCOSE:

SYMPTOMS:

DATE:

BP:

WEIGHT:

GLUCOSE:

SYMPTOMS:

DATE:

BP:

WEIGHT:

GLUCOSE:

SYMPTOMS:

DATE:

BP:

WEIGHT:

GLUCOSE:

SYMPTOMS:

DATE:

BP:

WEIGHT:

GLUCOSE:

SYMPTOMS:

DATE:

BP:

WEIGHT:

GLUCOSE:

SYMPTOMS:

DATE:

BP:

WEIGHT:

GLUCOSE:

SYMPTOMS:

DATE:

BP:

WEIGHT:

GLUCOSE:

SYMPTOMS:

DATE:

BP:

WEIGHT:

GLUCOSE:

SYMPTOMS:

DATE:

BP:

WEIGHT:

GLUCOSE:

SYMPTOMS:

DATE:

BP:

WEIGHT:

GLUCOSE:

SYMPTOMS:

DATE:

BP:

WEIGHT:

GLUCOSE:

SYMPTOMS:

DATE:

BP:

WEIGHT:

GLUCOSE:

SYMPTOMS:

DATE:

BP:

WEIGHT:

GLUCOSE:

SYMPTOMS:

DATE:

BP:

WEIGHT:

GLUCOSE:

SYMPTOMS:

DATE:

BP:

WEIGHT:

GLUCOSE:

SYMPTOMS:

DATE:

BP:

WEIGHT:

GLUCOSE:

SYMPTOMS:

DATE:

BP:

WEIGHT:

GLUCOSE:

SYMPTOMS:

DATE:

BP:

WEIGHT:

GLUCOSE:

SYMPTOMS:

DATE:

BP:

WEIGHT:

GLUCOSE:

SYMPTOMS:

DATE:

BP:

WEIGHT:

GLUCOSE:

SYMPTOMS:

DATE:

BP:

WEIGHT:

GLUCOSE:

SYMPTOMS:

DATE:

BP:

WEIGHT:

GLUCOSE:

SYMPTOMS:

DATE:

BP:

WEIGHT:

GLUCOSE:

SYMPTOMS:

DATE:

BP:

WEIGHT:

GLUCOSE:

SYMPTOMS:

DATE:

BP:

WEIGHT:

GLUCOSE:

SYMPTOMS:

DATE:

BP:

WEIGHT:

GLUCOSE:

SYMPTOMS:

DATE:

BP:

WEIGHT:

GLUCOSE:

SYMPTOMS:

DATE:

BP:

WEIGHT:

GLUCOSE:

SYMPTOMS:

DATE:

BP:

WEIGHT:

GLUCOSE:

SYMPTOMS:

DATE:

BP:

WEIGHT:

GLUCOSE:

SYMPTOMS:

DATE:

BP:

WEIGHT:

GLUCOSE:

SYMPTOMS:

DATE:

BP:

WEIGHT:

GLUCOSE:

SYMPTOMS:

DATE:

BP:

WEIGHT:

GLUCOSE:

SYMPTOMS:

DATE:

BP:

WEIGHT:

GLUCOSE:

SYMPTOMS:

DATE:

BP:

WEIGHT:

GLUCOSE:

SYMPTOMS:

DATE:

BP:

WEIGHT:

GLUCOSE:

SYMPTOMS:

DATE:

BP:

WEIGHT:

GLUCOSE:

SYMPTOMS:

DATE:

BP:

WEIGHT:

GLUCOSE:

SYMPTOMS:

DATE:

BP:

WEIGHT:

GLUCOSE:

SYMPTOMS:

DATE:

BP:

WEIGHT:

GLUCOSE:

SYMPTOMS:

DATE:

BP:

WEIGHT:

GLUCOSE:

SYMPTOMS:

DATE:

BP:

WEIGHT:

GLUCOSE:

SYMPTOMS:

DATE:

BP:

WEIGHT:

GLUCOSE:

SYMPTOMS:

DATE:

BP:

WEIGHT:

GLUCOSE:

SYMPTOMS:

DATE:

BP:

WEIGHT:

GLUCOSE:

SYMPTOMS:

DATE:

BP:

WEIGHT:

GLUCOSE:

SYMPTOMS:

DATE:

BP:

WEIGHT:

GLUCOSE:

SYMPTOMS:

DATE:

BP:

WEIGHT:

GLUCOSE:

SYMPTOMS:

DATE:

BP:

WEIGHT:

GLUCOSE:

SYMPTOMS:

DATE:

BP:

WEIGHT:

GLUCOSE:

SYMPTOMS:

DATE:

BP:

WEIGHT:

GLUCOSE:

SYMPTOMS:

DATE:

BP:

WEIGHT:

GLUCOSE:

SYMPTOMS:

DATE:

BP:

WEIGHT:

GLUCOSE:

SYMPTOMS:

DATE:

BP:

WEIGHT:

GLUCOSE:

SYMPTOMS:

DATE:

BP:

WEIGHT:

GLUCOSE:

SYMPTOMS:

DATE:

BP:

WEIGHT:

GLUCOSE:

SYMPTOMS:

DATE:

BP:

WEIGHT:

GLUCOSE:

SYMPTOMS:

DATE:

BP:

WEIGHT:

GLUCOSE:

SYMPTOMS:

DATE:

BP:

WEIGHT:

GLUCOSE:

SYMPTOMS:

DATE:

BP:

WEIGHT:

GLUCOSE:

SYMPTOMS:

DATE:

BP:

WEIGHT:

GLUCOSE:

SYMPTOMS:

DATE:

BP:

WEIGHT:

GLUCOSE:

SYMPTOMS:

DATE:

BP:

WEIGHT:

GLUCOSE:

SYMPTOMS:

DATE:

BP:

WEIGHT:

GLUCOSE:

SYMPTOMS:

DATE:

BP:

WEIGHT:

GLUCOSE:

SYMPTOMS:

DATE:

BP:

WEIGHT:

GLUCOSE:

SYMPTOMS:

DATE:

BP:

WEIGHT:

GLUCOSE:

SYMPTOMS:

DATE:

BP:

WEIGHT:

GLUCOSE:

SYMPTOMS:

DATE:

BP:

WEIGHT:

GLUCOSE:

SYMPTOMS:

DATE:

BP:

WEIGHT:

GLUCOSE:

SYMPTOMS:

DATE:

BP:

WEIGHT:

GLUCOSE:

SYMPTOMS:

DATE:

BP:

WEIGHT:

GLUCOSE:

SYMPTOMS:

DATE:

BP:

WEIGHT:

GLUCOSE:

SYMPTOMS:

DATE:

BP:

WEIGHT:

GLUCOSE:

SYMPTOMS:

DATE:

BP:

WEIGHT:

GLUCOSE:

SYMPTOMS:

DATE:

BP:

WEIGHT:

GLUCOSE:

SYMPTOMS:

DATE:

BP:

WEIGHT:

GLUCOSE:

SYMPTOMS:

DATE:

BP:

WEIGHT:

GLUCOSE:

SYMPTOMS:

DATE:

BP:

WEIGHT:

GLUCOSE:

SYMPTOMS:

DATE:

BP:

WEIGHT:

GLUCOSE:

SYMPTOMS:

DATE:

BP:

WEIGHT:

GLUCOSE:

SYMPTOMS:

DATE:

BP:

WEIGHT:

GLUCOSE:

SYMPTOMS:

DATE:

BP:

WEIGHT:

GLUCOSE:

SYMPTOMS:

DATE:

BP:

WEIGHT:

GLUCOSE:

SYMPTOMS:

DATE:

BP:

WEIGHT:

GLUCOSE:

SYMPTOMS:

DATE:

BP:

WEIGHT:

GLUCOSE:

SYMPTOMS:

DATE:

BP:

WEIGHT:

GLUCOSE:

SYMPTOMS:

DATE:

BP:

WEIGHT:

GLUCOSE:

SYMPTOMS:

DATE:

BP:

WEIGHT:

GLUCOSE:

SYMPTOMS:

DATE:

BP:

WEIGHT:

GLUCOSE:

SYMPTOMS:

DATE:

BP:

WEIGHT:

GLUCOSE:

SYMPTOMS:

DATE:

BP:

WEIGHT:

GLUCOSE:

SYMPTOMS:

DATE:

BP:

WEIGHT:

GLUCOSE:

SYMPTOMS:

DATE:

BP:

WEIGHT:

GLUCOSE:

SYMPTOMS:

DATE:

BP:

WEIGHT:

GLUCOSE:

SYMPTOMS:

DATE:

BP:

WEIGHT:

GLUCOSE:

SYMPTOMS:

DATE:

BP:

WEIGHT:

GLUCOSE:

SYMPTOMS:

DATE:

BP:

WEIGHT:

GLUCOSE:

SYMPTOMS:

DATE:

BP:

WEIGHT:

GLUCOSE:

SYMPTOMS:

DATE:

BP:

WEIGHT:

GLUCOSE:

SYMPTOMS:

DATE:

BP:

WEIGHT:

GLUCOSE:

SYMPTOMS:

DATE:

BP:

WEIGHT:

GLUCOSE:

SYMPTOMS:

DATE:

BP:

WEIGHT:

GLUCOSE:

SYMPTOMS:

DATE:

BP:

WEIGHT:

GLUCOSE:

SYMPTOMS:

DATE:

BP:

WEIGHT:

GLUCOSE:

SYMPTOMS:

DATE:

BP:

WEIGHT:

GLUCOSE:

SYMPTOMS:

DATE:

BP:

WEIGHT:

GLUCOSE:

SYMPTOMS:

DATE:

BP:

WEIGHT:

GLUCOSE:

SYMPTOMS:

DATE:

BP:

WEIGHT:

GLUCOSE:

SYMPTOMS:

DATE:

BP:

WEIGHT:

GLUCOSE:

SYMPTOMS:

DATE:

BP:

WEIGHT:

GLUCOSE:

SYMPTOMS:

DATE:

BP:

WEIGHT:

GLUCOSE:

SYMPTOMS:

DATE:

BP:

WEIGHT:

GLUCOSE:

SYMPTOMS:

DATE:

BP:

WEIGHT:

GLUCOSE:

SYMPTOMS:

DATE:

BP:

WEIGHT:

GLUCOSE:

SYMPTOMS:

DATE:

BP:

WEIGHT:

GLUCOSE:

SYMPTOMS:

DATE:

BP:

WEIGHT:

GLUCOSE:

SYMPTOMS:

DATE:

BP:

WEIGHT:

GLUCOSE:

SYMPTOMS:

DATE:

BP:

WEIGHT:

GLUCOSE:

SYMPTOMS:

DATE:

BP:

WEIGHT:

GLUCOSE:

SYMPTOMS:

DATE:

BP:

WEIGHT:

GLUCOSE:

SYMPTOMS:

DATE:

BP:

WEIGHT:

GLUCOSE:

SYMPTOMS:

DATE:

BP:

WEIGHT:

GLUCOSE:

SYMPTOMS:

DATE:

BP:

WEIGHT:

GLUCOSE:

SYMPTOMS:

DATE:

BP:

WEIGHT:

GLUCOSE:

SYMPTOMS:

DATE:

BP:

WEIGHT:

GLUCOSE:

SYMPTOMS:

DATE:

BP:

WEIGHT:

GLUCOSE:

SYMPTOMS:

DATE:

BP:

WEIGHT:

GLUCOSE:

SYMPTOMS:

DATE:

BP:

WEIGHT:

GLUCOSE:

SYMPTOMS:

DATE:

BP:

WEIGHT:

GLUCOSE:

SYMPTOMS:

DATE:

BP:

WEIGHT:

GLUCOSE:

SYMPTOMS:

DATE:

BP:

WEIGHT:

GLUCOSE:

SYMPTOMS:

DATE:

BP:

WEIGHT:

GLUCOSE:

SYMPTOMS:

DATE:

BP:

WEIGHT:

GLUCOSE:

SYMPTOMS:

DATE:

BP:

WEIGHT:

GLUCOSE:

SYMPTOMS: